CHRONIC PANCREATITIS MANAGEMENT DIET COOKBOOK

Nourishing Recipes For Healing And Relief:

Expert Guidance For Long Term Health

DR. SHAYLA LEWIS

CHAPTER ONE..10

Understanding Chronic Pancreatitis: An Overview..10

What is chronic pancreatitis? 10

Causes and risk factors. 11

Genetic factors: 11

Autoimmune conditions: 12

Chronic pancreatitis symptoms can range in severity and include 12

Importance of nutrition in treating symptoms..13

Low-fat diet: 13

Small, frequent meals 14

Nutrient-rich foods 14

Overview of the cookbook's methodology 15

Nutrition education: 15

Dietary guidelines: 16

Meal planning tools: 16

CHAPTER TWO 18

The role of nutrition in chronic pancreatitis management..18

How Nutrition Impacts Pancreatic Health 18

The Importance of A Balanced Diet 19

Nutrients to Focus On for Symptom Management 20

Foods to avoid or limit: 20

Balance Flavour and Nutrition in Recipes 21

Getting Started: Essential Kitchen Tools and Ingredients 22

Must-have kitchen tools for cooking with chronic pancreatitis 22

Blender or Food Processor: 22

Slow Cooker or Instant Pot 23

Food Scale: 23

Essential Ingredients for Nutritious Meals 24

Low-fat Protein Sources 24

Whole Grains 24

Good fats 25

Low-FODMAP Foods 25

Read Food Labels Carefully: 26

Stick to the periphery 26

Plan Ahead 26

Shop during off-peak hours:....................26

Meal Planning Strategies for Success:......27

Balanced Meals:....................................27

Hydration:..28

Easy Meal Preparation Techniques for
Busy Schedules.....................................28

Freezer-friendly Meals...........................28

Pre-cut and wash produce.....................29

Use Convenience Foods Wisely..............29

Understanding the Low-Carb, Antioxidant-
Rich, and Anti-Inflammatory Diet............30

Practical Strategies for Incorporating
These Diets into Everyday Meals..........30

Low-Carb Diets.....................................31

Antioxidant-Rich Diets...........................31

Anti-Inflammatory Diets:.........................32

The Advantages of Low-Carb Diets for
Pancreatitis Management.......................33

CHAPTER THREE....................................36

Antioxidants are important in reducing
inflammation...36

Foods with Anti-inflammatory Properties
....37

How These Diets Help Nerve Pain Relief.39

Practical Ways to Incorporate These Diets into Your Everyday Meals...........41

Focus on entire, unprocessed foods: 41

Choose healthy cooking methods...........42

Plan ahead: 43

Chronic Pancreatitis Management Diet Cookbook 43

Recipe Modification Ideas: 44

How to Adapt Recipes to Meet Your Dietary Needs 44

Substitute Ingredients for Healthier Options: 45

Reducing Fat Content without sacrificing Flavor...46

Managing Portion Size for Optimal Digestion: 46

Cooking Techniques That Improve Nutrient Absorption 47

Introduction: 48

Low-carb breakfast options for sustained energy:...48

Antioxidant-rich breakfast recipes:.......49

Tips for Quick and Easy Breakfast Preparation 50

CHAPTER FOUR 52

Nourishing Soups and Salads: Light and Filling Meals 52

Healing Soups Full of Nutrients 52

Salad Recipes with a Refreshing Boost 54

Anti-inflammatory dressings and toppings. 55

Tips for Creating Filling and Gentle Meals 56

CHAPTER FIVE 58

How to customize soups and salads to your liking 58

Flavorful main dishes are satisfying and nutritious 59

Low-carb entrees to keep you satisfied .61

Antioxidant-rich ingredients for taste and health 63

Anti-inflammatory Spices & Herbs 65

CHAPTER SIX 68

Cooking Techniques that Preserve Nutrients 68

Healthy Side Dishes to Complement Any Meal 73

Snack Options for On-the-Go Nutrition 74

Snacks Packed with Antioxidants for Long-Lasting Energy..75

Portion Control Strategies for Snacking Success 76

Sweet Treats: Indulge Without Guilt 77

CHAPTER SEVEN 80

Tips for Mindful Dessert Enjoyment.....80

Balancing Sweetness and Healthfulness..80

Nourishing recipes and expert advice for long-term management of chronic pancreatitis 81

Ginger Turmeric Smoothie: 81

Quinoa Vegetable Soup 81

Banana Oat Pancakes: 82

A 30-day meal plan to alleviate symptoms, promote healing, and cultivate optimal pancreatic wellness. ..83

THE END 85

DISCLAIMER

Write a brief complete Disclaimer for my diet cook book telling them that the author is not in any association with any company, business or individual and also this book is written by the authors knowledge and understanding

The information provided in this diet cookbook is based on the author's personal knowledge and understanding. The author is not affiliated with, endorsed by, or associated with any company, business, or individual. The recipes and dietary advice contained within this book are intended for informational purposes only. Readers should consult with a healthcare professional or a registered dietitian before making any significant changes to their diet or lifestyle. The author assumes no responsibility for any adverse effects that may result from the use or misuse of the information contained in this book.

CHAPTER ONE

Understanding Chronic Pancreatitis: An Overview

Chronic pancreatitis is a long-term inflammation of the pancreas that frequently causes irreversible damage and impairment of its function. This illness progresses gradually over time, with repeated bouts of inflammation generating scarring and fibrosis in the pancreatic tissue. Chronic pancreatitis, as opposed to acute pancreatitis, is a long-term illness that can have a major influence on a person's quality of life.

What is chronic pancreatitis?

Chronic pancreatitis is defined as prolonged inflammation of the pancreas, a gland located behind the stomach. The pancreas is important for digestion and blood sugar management because it produces digestive enzymes and hormones like insulin. persistent pancreatitis causes inflammation of the pancreatic tissue, which leads to consequences such as nutrient malabsorption, diabetes, and persistent discomfort.

Causes and risk factors.

The precise etiology of chronic pancreatitis is frequently unknown, however, various factors can contribute to its development:

Alcohol abuse: Heavy and sustained alcohol drinking is a major cause of chronic pancreatitis. Alcohol destroys pancreatic tissue, causing inflammation and scarring over time.

Cigarette smoking raises the likelihood of developing chronic pancreatitis. Tobacco's toxic compounds can injure the pancreas and aggravate inflammation.

Genetic factors: Some people inherit genetic alterations that predispose them to pancreatic illnesses such as chronic pancreatitis.

Gallstones, pancreatic tumors, and anatomical anomalies can block the pancreatic ducts, causing digestive enzyme buildup and subsequent inflammation.

Autoimmune conditions: Autoimmune pancreatitis is a rare type of chronic pancreatitis in which the immune system incorrectly targets pancreatic tissue, resulting in inflammation.

Symptoms and diagnoses

Chronic pancreatitis symptoms can range in severity and include:

Chronic pancreatitis is characterized by persistent or recurring discomfort in the upper abdomen, which can radiate to the back.

Poor nutrient absorption can cause weight loss, diarrhea, and greasy stools (steatorrhea).

Digestive enzyme abnormalities can lead to nausea, vomiting, and reduced appetite.

Damage to insulin-producing cells in the pancreas can cause diabetes mellitus.

Obstructed pancreatic ducts can cause jaundice, a yellowing of the skin and eyes.

Chronic pancreatitis is normally diagnosed using a combination of medical history, physical examination, imaging testing (such as a CT scan or MRI), and pancreatic function tests.

Importance of nutrition in treating symptoms

Diet is critical in treating the symptoms of chronic pancreatitis and enhancing the quality of life for those living with the condition. A well-balanced diet helps reduce stomach pain, avoid malnutrition, and improve pancreatic function. Key dietary factors for managing chronic pancreatitis include:

Low-fat diet: Because the pancreas creates digestive enzymes to break down fats, limiting fat intake can reduce the pancreas' workload and improve digestive symptoms.

Small, frequent meals: Eating smaller meals throughout the day can help minimize pancreatic overstimulation and lower the likelihood of experiencing pain or discomfort.

Limiting alcohol and caffeine: Because alcohol and caffeine can irritate the pancreas and worsen inflammation, it is critical to restrict or avoid these drugs.

Nutrient-rich foods: Eating nutrient-dense foods like fruits, vegetables, lean proteins, and whole grains will help you get enough vitamins and minerals while reducing digestive stress.

Hydration: Staying hydrated is essential for maintaining proper digestion and avoiding issues like dehydration or electrolyte imbalance.

A certified dietitian can make personalized dietary recommendations based on an individual's needs, tastes, and nutritional status.

Overview of the cookbook's methodology

The Chronic Pancreatitis Management Diet Cookbook provides a complete approach to treating chronic pancreatitis using dietary treatments. This cookbook aims to help people with chronic pancreatitis make informed eating choices that benefit their health and well-being. Key elements of the cookbook's methodology include:

Nutrition education: The cookbook contains thorough information regarding the significance of diet in managing chronic pancreatitis, such as meal planning, item replacements, and quantity control.

Recipe selection: The cookbook includes a variety of delicious and nutritious meals that are specifically targeted to the nutritional demands of people with chronic pancreatitis. These recipes emphasize low-fat, nutrient-dense ingredients and use flavor-enhancing techniques to make meals delightful and rewarding.

Dietary guidelines: The cookbook provides practical dietary advice and recommendations for treating chronic pancreatitis symptoms, including which foods to include or avoid. It also addresses basic dietary concerns, such as getting enough protein, managing diabetes, and avoiding nutritional deficiencies.

Meal planning tools: The cookbook contains meal planning templates, grocery lists, and culinary ideas to help users make dietary changes and prepare pancreatitis-friendly meals at home.

Support resources: In addition to recipes and meal plans, the cookbook may include nutritional information tables, culinary techniques, and lifestyle advice to assist people with chronic pancreatitis in achieving and maintaining optimal health outcomes.

Overall, the Chronic Pancreatitis Control Diet Cookbook is an excellent resource for anyone looking for practical advice and delicious dishes to help them on their journey to better health and symptom control. Individuals with chronic pancreatitis can use the cookbook's approach to improve their nutritional condition, reduce symptoms, and improve their general quality of life.

CHAPTER TWO

The role of nutrition in chronic pancreatitis management

Nutrition is critical in the treatment of chronic pancreatitis, which is characterized by long-term pancreatic inflammation. Given the pancreas' vital responsibilities in digestion and blood sugar management, food choices have a substantial impact on its health and function. Individuals with chronic pancreatitis can benefit from a personalized diet that reduces symptoms, supports pancreatic function, and improves general well-being.

How Nutrition Impacts Pancreatic Health:

The effects of nutrition on pancreatic health are diverse. Certain dietary components can either worsen inflammation and pancreatic damage or help to cure and relieve symptoms. For example, excessive fat consumption, particularly saturated and trans fats, might cause pancreatic enzyme release, resulting in further inflammation and pain. On the other hand, a diet high in antioxidants, and fiber, and low in processed foods can help minimize oxidative stress, inflammation, and pancreatic strain.

The Importance of A Balanced Diet

A well-balanced diet is essential in chronic pancreatitis care for a variety of reasons. For starters, it guarantees that important elements like vitamins, minerals, protein, and healthy fats are consumed in sufficient amounts for overall health and healing. Second, a well-balanced diet helps to maintain blood sugar levels, avoiding issues related to pancreatic dysfunction, such as diabetes. Finally, it promotes digestive health by providing sufficient fiber and water, which aid in nutrition absorption and stool regularity.

In chronic pancreatitis, focusing on specific nutrients can help relieve symptoms and promote pancreatic function. For example, eating lean protein sources such as poultry, fish, and tofu can offer needed amino acids without overstimulating pancreatic enzymes. Consuming antioxidant-rich foods including fruits, vegetables, nuts, and seeds can also help reduce inflammation and oxidative stress. Furthermore, emphasizing complex carbohydrates and fiber can help with digestion and reduce blood sugar rise.

Foods to avoid or limit:

Certain meals might worsen symptoms and should be avoided or limited in chronic pancreatitis care. High-fat diets, fried foods, processed meats, and rich desserts can overwhelm the pancreas, causing inflammation and pain. Furthermore, alcohol use should be severely controlled or avoided entirely, as it can directly damage pancreatic tissue and worsen symptoms. Spicy foods and caffeine may also cause pain in certain people, so they should be consumed in moderation.

Balance Flavour and Nutrition in Recipes

Developing delectable yet healthful foods for people with chronic pancreatitis needs ingenuity and careful planning. Instead of frying, choose baking, grilling, or steaming to reduce fat content while maintaining flavor. Using herbs, spices, citrus zest, and vinegar can improve flavor without relying on too much salt or sugar. A variety of colorful fruits and vegetables not only offer visual appeal, but also contain critical vitamins, minerals, and antioxidants. Experimenting with different ingredients and cooking methods can help you create a balance between flavor and nutrition, resulting in pleasurable meals that promote pancreatic health.

Getting Started: Essential Kitchen Tools and Ingredients

Living with chronic pancreatitis demands meticulous food preparation and planning. Establishing a well-equipped kitchen and stocking up on the necessary materials are critical steps toward effectively controlling this disease.

Must-have kitchen tools for cooking with chronic pancreatitis:

Nonstick Cookware: Investing in high-quality nonstick cookware can dramatically eliminate the need for extra fats or oils while cooking, which is especially advantageous for pancreatitis patients who need to limit their fat consumption.

Blender or Food Processor: These gadgets are essential for achieving smooth textures, particularly for making pureed dishes or blending fruits and vegetables into soups and sauces.

Sharp Knives: A set of sharp knives makes chopping and slicing simpler and safer. Dull blades can cause uneven slices, requiring additional cooking time and affecting the dish's overall texture.

Slow Cooker or Instant Pot: These kitchen appliances are perfect for making fragrant, tender meals with little effort. Slow cooking allows for slow, progressive cooking, which can improve the flavor and digestibility of dishes for people with pancreatitis.

Food Scale: Precise portion control is essential for treating pancreatitis symptoms, particularly fat consumption. A food scale ensures accurate measures, allowing people to follow dietary requirements more efficiently.

Steamer Basket: Steaming is a healthy cooking method that retains nutrients and natural flavors in foods. A steamer basket is ideal for cooking vegetables, fish, and other delicate items without adding grease.

Essential Ingredients for Nutritious Meals

Low-fat Protein Sources: Choose lean meats such as chicken, turkey, and fish, as well as plant-based proteins like tofu and lentils. Protein is necessary for tissue repair and muscle maintenance, however, those with pancreatitis should eat lean foods to reduce fat intake.

Whole Grains: Incorporate whole grains such as quinoa, brown rice, and whole wheat pasta into your meals for long-lasting energy and fiber, which promotes digestion and prevents constipation—a typical problem for people with pancreatitis.

Good fats: While fat consumption should be limited, it is critical to incorporate small amounts of good fats into the diet, such as olive oil, avocado, and almonds. These fats include necessary fatty acids and promote satiety without worsening pancreatitis symptoms.

Low-FODMAP Foods: Some people with chronic pancreatitis may benefit from eating a low-FODMAP diet, which limits specific carbs that might cause digestive problems. Rice, oats, lactose-free dairy products, and various fruits and vegetables are popular low-FODMAP pantry staples.

Herbs and spices like ginger, turmeric, cinnamon, and parsley can help to improve the flavor of dishes without adding too much salt or fat. These compounds include antioxidants and may have anti-inflammatory qualities, which might help manage pancreatitis.

Tips for Shopping With Chronic Pancreatitis:

Read Food Labels Carefully: Check food labels for ingredients high in fat, sugar, and additives, which might cause pancreatitis symptoms. When feasible, look for items with the labels "low-fat," "reduced sodium," and "no added sugar".

Stick to the periphery: When shopping at the grocery store, focus on the periphery, where fresh vegetables, lean proteins, and dairy items are usually found. Spend less time in the processed food aisles, where tempting but potentially dangerous goods abound.

Plan Ahead: Before going to the store, develop a list of what you need and stick to it to prevent making impulse purchases. Planning your meals for the week might help you save time and money on groceries.

Shop during off-peak hours: Crowded grocery stores can be overwhelming, especially for those with chronic pancreatitis, who may require extra time to read labels and compare items. Shop during less busy hours to reduce stress and make the experience more enjoyable.

Meal Planning Strategies for Success:

Balanced Meals: Aim to prepare meals that contain lean protein, complex carbohydrates, and plenty of veggies. Eating equally throughout the day can help regulate blood sugar levels and minimize stomach pain.

Portion Control: Watch your portion amounts to avoid overeating, which can strain the pancreas and increase symptoms. Using smaller dishes and measuring servings with a food scale can help with portion control.

Instead of three substantial meals, try eating smaller, more regular meals throughout the day. This method can assist to avoid overwhelming the digestive system and may ease symptoms such as bloating and stomach pain.

Hydration: Stay well-hydrated by drinking plenty of water throughout the day. Dehydration can exacerbate pancreatitis symptoms, so aim to drink at least eight glasses of water each day, or more if necessary, particularly in hot weather or after physical exertion.

Easy Meal Preparation Techniques for Busy Schedules

Batch Cooking: Set aside a day or two every week to batch-cook staple components such as grains, proteins, and veggies. Preparing these ingredients ahead of time saves time during the week and enables speedy meal assembly when time is of the essence.

Freezer-friendly Meals: Make soups, stews, and casseroles in bulk and divide them into individual servings for simple warming. This guarantees that you always have a nutritious supper on hand, even on busy days.

Pre-cut and wash produce: As soon as you arrive home from the store, wash and chop fruits and vegetables to make them ready for snacking or dinner preparation. Preparing veggies in advance saves time when cooking later in the week.

Use Convenience Foods Wisely: Although complete, unprocessed foods are preferable, there are instances when convenience foods can be useful. To simplify meal preparation while maintaining nutrition, select for low-fat, low-sodium products such as pre-cooked grains, canned beans, and pre-cut vegetables.

You can effectively manage chronic pancreatitis and enjoy delicious, nourishing meals that support your overall health and well-being by stocking your kitchen with essential tools and nutritious ingredients, implementing meal planning strategies, and incorporating simple meal prep techniques into your routine.

Understanding the Low-Carb, Antioxidant-Rich, and Anti-Inflammatory Diet

Advantages of Low-Carb Diets for Pancreatitis Management

Antioxidants are important for reducing inflammation.

Foods with Anti-Inflammatory Properties

How These Diets Help Nerve Pain Relief

Understanding low-carb, antioxidant-rich, and anti-inflammatory diets:

Chronic pancreatitis is a disorder characterized by pancreatic inflammation, which can cause stomach pain, digestive problems, and, in some cases, malnutrition. Dietary changes can help relieve discomfort and enhance overall health. In this context, three important dietary methods include low-carb, antioxidant-rich, and anti-inflammatory diets.

Low-Carb Diets: These diets focus on lowering carbs, particularly refined sugars and starches. By limiting carbohydrate intake, blood sugar levels remain steady, putting less burden on the pancreas to create insulin. This stability can help manage symptoms such as stomach pain and digestive discomfort, which are prevalent with pancreatitis. Low-carb diets are also known to encourage weight loss, which helps relieve pancreatic strain and increase insulin sensitivity.

Antioxidant-Rich Diets: Antioxidants are molecules found in foods that help neutralize damaging free radicals in the body, which can cause inflammation and tissue damage. In the setting of pancreatitis, antioxidants have an important role in decreasing inflammation in the pancreas and other organs. Consuming foods high in antioxidants, such as fruits, vegetables, nuts, and seeds, can help protect pancreatic cells and improve overall pancreatic health.

Anti-Inflammatory Diets: Chronic inflammation is a typical component of pancreatitis, which can worsen symptoms and complications. Anti-inflammatory diets focus on eating foods that help to reduce inflammation in the body. This usually entails integrating omega-3 fatty acids, which are found in fatty fish like salmon and flaxseeds, as well as foods strong in fiber and phytonutrients, such as leafy greens, blueberries, and turmeric. These diets, which reduce inflammatory triggers and promote a balanced inflammatory response, can help ease symptoms and enhance overall well-being.

The Advantages of Low-Carb Diets for Pancreatitis Management

Low-carb diets provide various advantages for those with chronic pancreatitis. For starters, by lowering carbohydrate intake, these diets help stabilize blood sugar levels, which is critical for pancreatic health and insulin regulation. Stable blood sugar levels can help relieve symptoms like stomach pain and digestive discomfort that are prevalent with pancreatitis.

Furthermore, low-carb diets frequently result in weight loss, which might be advantageous to people with pancreatitis. Excess weight puts an additional burden on the pancreas, which can worsen inflammation and insulin resistance. Low-carb diets, which promote weight loss, can help minimize this burden while also enhancing pancreatic function and overall health.

Furthermore, low-carb diets may improve lipid profiles by lowering triglyceride levels, which are commonly increased in people with pancreatitis. High triglyceride levels can cause inflammation and raise the risk of consequences including pancreatitis attacks. Low-carb diets, which lower triglycerides, can help reduce these risks and improve disease management.

Overall, low-carb diets for pancreatitis care offer improved blood sugar control, weight loss, and lower triglyceride levels, all of which lead to better symptom management and pancreatic health.

CHAPTER THREE

Antioxidants are important in reducing inflammation

Antioxidants help to reduce inflammation, which is a major contributor to the progression and severity of chronic pancreatitis. Pancreatic inflammation can cause tissue damage, discomfort, and consequences including pancreatic insufficiency and diabetes. Antioxidants protect pancreatic cells and tissues from damage by neutralizing free radicals and lowering oxidative stress, hence moderating inflammation and its effects.

Plant-based foods like fruits, vegetables, nuts, and seeds are excellent providers of antioxidants. These foods contain a variety of antioxidants, including vitamins C and E, beta-carotene, and polyphenols, all of which have been found to reduce inflammation. Additionally, certain spices and herbs, such as turmeric, ginger, and cinnamon, are high in antioxidants and can be added to the diet to boost their anti-inflammatory properties.

Individuals with chronic pancreatitis can reduce inflammation, relieve symptoms, and enhance pancreatic function by including antioxidant-rich foods in their diet. Furthermore, antioxidants have been linked to a lower incidence of complications such as pancreatic cancer, emphasizing their significance in long-term illness management.

Foods with Anti-inflammatory Properties
Inflammation is a typical component of chronic pancreatitis, and it can worsen symptoms and complications. However, several foods have anti-inflammatory characteristics and can help reduce inflammation throughout the body, including the pancreas. Incorporating these foods into

your diet can help with symptom management and overall pancreatic health.

Fatty fish like salmon, mackerel, and sardines contain omega-3 fatty acids, which have powerful anti-inflammatory properties. These fatty acids aid in preventing inflammation by limiting the formation of pro-inflammatory chemicals in the body.

Fruits and vegetables are also rich in anti-inflammatory components such as vitamins, minerals, and phytonutrients. Berries, cherries, oranges, kale, spinach, and broccoli are especially high in antioxidants and anti-inflammatory chemicals.

Nuts and seeds, such as almonds, walnuts, flaxseeds, and chia seeds, are high in omega-3 fatty acids, fiber, and antioxidants, all of which help to reduce inflammation.

Furthermore, herbs and spices such as turmeric, ginger, garlic, and cinnamon contain bioactive components with anti-inflammatory qualities that can be utilized to flavor dishes while also increasing their nutritional value.

Individuals suffering from chronic pancreatitis can reduce inflammation, alleviate symptoms, and enhance overall pancreatic health by including these anti-inflammatory foods in their diet.

How These Diets Help Nerve Pain Relief

Chronic pancreatitis is frequently associated with neuropathic pain, which can be debilitating and difficult to treat. Low-carb, antioxidant-rich, and anti-inflammatory diets, on the other hand, have a number of mechanisms that can help people with chronic pancreatitis relieve nerve pain and enhance their overall health.

For starters, low-carb diets help stabilize blood sugar levels, which can minimize nerve damage and neuropathic discomfort caused by diabetic neuropathy. These diets help prevent nerve damage and relieve symptoms like burning, tingling, and numbness by reducing blood sugar fluctuations.

Second, antioxidants protect nerves from oxidative stress and inflammation, both of which cause nerve pain. Antioxidants aid in the preservation of nerve function and relief of neuropathic pain associated with chronic pancreatitis by neutralizing free radicals and decreasing inflammation.

Finally, anti-inflammatory foods help lower inflammation throughout the body, including the nerves, which can aid with neuropathic pain. These diets aid in pain relief and nerve health by reducing inflammatory triggers and supporting a balanced inflammatory response.

Overall, low-carb, antioxidant-rich, and anti-inflammatory diets can help people with chronic pancreatitis relieve nerve pain and enhance their quality of life through a variety of mechanisms.

Practical Ways to Incorporate These Diets into Your Everyday Meals

Incorporating low-carb, antioxidant-rich, and anti-inflammatory diets into daily meals may appear difficult at first, but with proper planning and ingenuity, it can be both delicious and enjoyable. Here are some practical strategies for implementing these diets into your daily meals.

Focus on entire, unprocessed foods: Plan your meals around whole foods like fruits, vegetables, lean meats, and healthy fats.

Reduce your consumption of processed and refined foods, which are generally heavy in carbs but lacking in nutrients.

Experiment with new recipes: Try out new recipes that use antioxidant-rich items like berries, leafy greens, nuts, and seeds. Look for recipes with lean proteins like fish and chicken, as well as healthy fats like avocado and olive oil.

Aim to fill half of your plate with colorful fruits and vegetables at each meal. Different colors represent different antioxidants, therefore using a variety of colors guarantees that you obtain a diverse spectrum of nutrients and antioxidants.

Choose healthy cooking methods: Steaming, baking, grilling, and sautéing are all good options for preserving the nutritional value of foods. Avoid frying and deep-frying, which can add extra calories and bad fats to your food.

Experiment using herbs and spices to add flavor to your meals without relying on salt, sugar, or bad fats. Examples include turmeric, ginger, garlic, and cinnamon.

Plan ahead: Set aside some time each week to plan your meals and snacks, ensuring that you include a variety of nutrient-dense foods that will help you achieve your dietary objectives. This will allow you to stay on schedule and avoid making poor choices when hunger strikes.

Following these practical guidelines and including low-carb, antioxidant-rich, and anti-inflammatory foods in your daily meals will help you manage pancreatitis while also improving your general health and well-being.

Chronic Pancreatitis Management Diet Cookbook:

Chronic pancreatitis necessitates strict dietary control to reduce symptoms and improve healing. A cookbook specifically designed for this illness can be an invaluable resource, providing tips on dish modification, product replacement, portion management, and cooking techniques:

Recipe Modification Ideas: Making Your Favorite Meals Pancreatitis-Friendly

Living with chronic pancreatitis should not mean giving up on wonderful food. Instead, it entails strategically modifying recipes to make them easier on the pancreas yet remaining fulfilling. This section of the cookbook would most likely provide detailed guidance on how to modify existing dishes to make them pancreatitis-friendly. It may contain recommendations such as lowering fat content, decreasing spice use, and emphasizing nutrient-dense products.

How to Adapt Recipes to Meet Your Dietary Needs:

Every person's nutritional demands are unique, and people with chronic pancreatitis frequently have specific requirements. This chapter will provide information on customizing recipes to accommodate varied dietary constraints and preferences. It may discuss gluten-free, low-fat, low-sugar, or low-fiber modifications, allowing readers to customize recipes to their specific needs without sacrificing taste or nutrition.

Substitute Ingredients for Healthier Options:
Ingredient substitution is an essential part of adjusting recipes for pancreatitis management. This section will look into healthier alternatives to common components

that can exacerbate pancreatic inflammation or discomfort. For example, replace saturated fats with healthier fats such as olive oil or avocado oil, use whole grains instead of processed grains, and choose lean meats over fatty cuts of meat.

Reducing Fat Content without sacrificing Flavor

Fat restriction is typically necessary in the treatment of chronic pancreatitis, but it does not have to mean bland or unappealing food. This section of the cookbook would go over inventive ways to minimize fat while increasing flavor using herbs, spices, and other seasonings. Roasting, grilling, and steaming can enhance the flavor of dishes without relying excessively on added fats.

Managing Portion Size for Optimal Digestion: Portion control is important in reducing the digestive stress on the pancreas. This chapter will provide practical ideas for establishing optimal portion sizes as well as practices for mindful eating. Smaller, more frequent meals and nutrient-dense foods might help you stay energized while minimizing discomfort.

Cooking Techniques That Improve Nutrient Absorption

Individuals with chronic pancreatitis require proper vitamin absorption because malabsorption can increase symptoms and cause nutritional deficits. This chapter will highlight cooking methods that improve nutritional bioavailability, such as lightly boiling vegetables to retain vitamins and minerals or combining particular foods to increase absorption, such as ingesting vitamin C-rich foods with iron sources.

In essence, a Chronic Pancreatitis Control Diet Cookbook would be an invaluable resource for people dealing with the issues of dietary control. By providing practical suggestions on recipe modification, food replacement, portion control, and cooking techniques, readers are empowered to take charge of their diet while also boosting pancreatic health and general well-being.

Breakfast Delights: Starting Your Day Right

Introduction: Breakfast is frequently regarded as the most crucial meal of the day, particularly for individuals suffering from chronic pancreatitis. Starting your day with a nutritious and balanced meal can set the tone for the rest of the day by giving long-lasting energy and critical nutrients. In this section of the Chronic Pancreatitis Management Diet Cookbook, we focus on creating tasty breakfast options that not only satisfy your taste buds but also help you achieve your health goals.

Low-carb breakfast options for sustained energy: A low-carb diet can help those with chronic pancreatitis by reducing strain on the pancreas and reducing symptoms like abdominal pain. We've compiled a list of low-carbohydrate breakfast recipes that nevertheless provide the nutrition you need to get through the day. These dishes use items like eggs, lean proteins, healthy fats, and fiber-rich veggies to keep you satisfied and energized without generating blood sugar spikes.

Antioxidant-rich breakfast recipes: Antioxidants help to reduce inflammation and oxidative stress, both of which are major symptoms of chronic pancreatitis. Our breakfast recipes feature antioxidant-rich nutrients including berries, nuts, seeds, and leafy greens. These components not only offer brilliant flavors and colors to your breakfast, but they also contain critical nutrients that promote your general health and well-being.

Anti-inflammatory substances for pain relief: Chronic pancreatitis is frequently associated with prolonged pain and discomfort. Incorporating anti-inflammatory items into your breakfast can help reduce symptoms and encourage healing. Turmeric, ginger, garlic, and fatty fish are examples of substances with anti-inflammatory effects that we include in our recipes. These components not only enhance the flavor of your meals but also help with your overall pain management plan.

Tips for Quick and Easy Breakfast Preparation

We understand how hectic mornings can be, especially when dealing with chronic pancreatitis. That's why we've included useful ideas and tactics for quick and easy breakfast preparation. From meal planning supplies ahead of time to using kitchen gadgets for speedy cooking, these ideas can help you streamline your morning routine and guarantee that you always have a nutritious breakfast ready to eat.

Meal options to suit different tastes and preferences: Variety is essential for keeping a healthy and enjoyable diet, especially when dealing with a chronic ailment like pancreatitis. Our breakfast section has a variety of food options to accommodate different tastes and preferences. Whether you prefer savory omelets, sweet smoothie bowls, or hefty breakfast hashes, you'll find something to please your appetite and replenish your body.

Finally, the Breakfast Delights portion of the Chronic Pancreatitis Management Diet Cookbook offers detailed guidance to getting your day started with tasty and nutritious breakfast selections. From low-carb meals for prolonged energy to anti-inflammatory substances for pain relief, we have everything you need to support your health and well-being while you work to manage chronic pancreatitis.

CHAPTER FOUR

Nourishing Soups and Salads: Light and Filling Meals

Chronic pancreatitis management frequently involves a careful dietary strategy, with an emphasis on nourishing, moderate foods that supply important nutrients without increasing symptoms. Soups and salads are ideal alternatives in this regard since they provide diversity, hydration, and a variety of vitamins and minerals that are essential for good health. Let's look at the ideas behind creating a chronic pancreatitis-friendly cookbook section devoted to these light yet delicious meals.

Soups are a comfortable staple in the diet of those with chronic pancreatitis. They provide an easy way to ingest critical nutrients while staying hydrated. When creating soup recipes for chronic pancreatitis, it's important to prioritize components that are both easy to digest and nutrient-packed. Choose lean proteins such as chicken or turkey, which supply essential amino acids without overloading the digestive system with lipids. Carrots, spinach, and zucchini are good sources of vitamins and fiber while still being soft on the stomach.

Incorporating medicinal herbs and spices such as ginger and turmeric can boost the nutritional value of soups while also delivering anti-inflammatory benefits. These ingredients have qualities that may help relieve pancreatic symptoms including discomfort and inflammation. Furthermore, using homemade, low-sodium broths or stocks as a basis gives you more control over the soup's flavor and sodium content, which is especially important for people with pancreatitis.

Salad Recipes with a Refreshing Boost

Salads are a refreshing and customizable choice for people who have chronic pancreatitis. When developing salad recipes for this audience, prioritize components that are both hydrating and easy on the digestive system. Leafy greens, such as spinach, romaine lettuce, and kale, contain critical vitamins and minerals while being low in fiber, making them easy to digest. Adding hydrating fruits like cucumbers, tomatoes, and berries can improve the salad's nutritional value and flavor profile.

Incorporating lean proteins such as grilled chicken or tofu increases fullness without overwhelming the digestive system. Individuals with chronic pancreatitis benefit from eating lean protein sources since it reduces discomfort and the danger of triggering symptoms. Furthermore, consuming healthy fats like avocado, nuts, and seeds can deliver necessary nutrients while also increasing feelings of fullness and satisfaction.

Anti-inflammatory dressings and toppings.

The primary goal of managing chronic pancreatitis is to reduce inflammation. Making dressings and toppings with anti-inflammatory ingredients can assist achieve this goal while also adding flavor and texture to soups and salads. Extra virgin olive oil, apple cider vinegar, and fresh herbs such as basil and parsley are all anti-inflammatory and can be combined to make delightful sauces and toppings.

When preparing recipes for those who have chronic pancreatitis, it is critical to avoid items high in saturated fats, processed sugars, and artificial additives. Instead, use whole ingredients and natural flavor enhancers to make dressings and toppings that support healing and overall health.

Tips for Creating Filling and Gentle Meals

When creating soups and salads for chronic pancreatitis care, it is critical to create a balance between nutrition and tenderness. Incorporating a range of textures, flavors, and nutrient-dense products ensures that meals are enjoyable without causing discomfort or increasing symptoms.

Including complex carbohydrate sources such as quinoa, brown rice, or sweet potatoes can help deliver long-lasting energy without overwhelming the digestive system. These components also help to increase feelings of fullness, which promotes post-meal contentment.

Furthermore, adding protein-rich items such as beans, eggs, or lean meats can aid in muscle maintenance and regeneration without overburdening the digestive system. Protein intake can be divided throughout the day and combined with fiber-rich foods such as vegetables and whole grains to help digestion and nutrient absorption.

CHAPTER FIVE

How to customize soups and salads to your liking

Customization is essential in managing chronic pancreatitis since it allows for individual preferences and dietary needs. Recipe versatility allows people to customize their meals while yet being mild on the digestive system.

Offering a wide range of soup bases, protein alternatives, and vegetable combinations provides for limitless customization opportunities. Providing suggestions for food substitutions and alternative flavor profiles allows people to experiment with new combinations while staying within their dietary constraints.

When customizing soups and salads for chronic pancreatitis care, it is crucial to encourage consciousness about portion amounts and meal frequency. Eating smaller, more frequent meals can assist in avoiding overloading the digestive system and reduce the likelihood of triggering symptoms.

Flavorful main dishes are satisfying and nutritious

When preparing delectable main courses for people with chronic pancreatitis, it is critical to establish a balance between taste and nutrition. These foods should not only satisfy the palate but also supply important nutrients that promote general health and well-being. Using a variety of ingredients, textures, and flavors can help make meals more interesting and pleasurable.

Consider meals with lean proteins like poultry, fish, and tofu, which are easier to digest and less likely to worsen pancreatitis symptoms. Incorporating a variety of vegetables, whole grains, and legumes into the diet increases fiber, vitamins, and minerals, improving digestive health and delivering critical nutrients.

Experiment with different cooking techniques to bring out the natural flavors of ingredients without relying on extra fats or sweets. Grilling, roasting, and sautéing can enhance the natural sweetness and depth of vegetables and proteins, whilst steaming and poaching preserve moisture and suppleness.

Don't be afraid to experiment with herbs, spices, and aromatics to improve the flavor of your dishes. Fresh herbs like basil, cilantro, and parsley can provide brightness and freshness, whereas spices like ginger, turmeric, and cumin provide depth and warmth. Citrus zest and juices can also add acidity and brightness to help balance flavors.

Finally, tasty main dishes for chronic pancreatitis management should prioritize whole, minimally processed products while paying attention to portion amounts and overall dietary balance.

A low-carb diet can assist people with chronic pancreatitis relieve symptoms and promote greater pancreatic health. Low-carb dinners emphasize high-quality proteins, healthy fats, and fiber-rich veggies while limiting refined carbohydrates and sugar consumption.

Explore dishes that use spiralized veggies, cauliflower rice, and lettuce wraps instead of carb-heavy foods like pasta, rice, and bread. These alternatives not only cut carbohydrate intake but also improve nutrient density.

Incorporate lean proteins such as chicken, turkey, fish, and plant-based sources such as tofu and tempeh to give satiety without putting further strain on the pancreas. Fatty fish, such as salmon and mackerel, include omega-3 fatty acids, which are anti-inflammatory and promote pancreatic health.

Include a variety of non-starchy veggies in your diet, such as leafy greens, broccoli, bell peppers, and zucchini, to offer volume, fiber, and vital nutrients. These vegetables are low in carbohydrates but abundant in nutrients, making them excellent alternatives for people with chronic pancreatitis.

Experiment with tasty sauces and dressings created from healthy fats such as olive oil, avocado, and almonds to improve the taste and texture of low-carb meals. Herbs, spices, and citrus can also enhance the flavor and complexity of recipes without the need for extra sugars or salt.

Individuals with chronic pancreatitis can enjoy fulfilling meals while improving their overall health and well-being by focusing on low-carb dinners high in protein, fiber, and healthy fats.

Antioxidant-rich ingredients for taste and health

Individuals with chronic pancreatitis should incorporate antioxidant-rich components into their diet since these compounds help reduce inflammation, protect against oxidative stress, and support pancreatic health. Include a range of antioxidant-rich fruits, vegetables, nuts, seeds, and spices in your meals to improve both the flavor and nutritional content.

Choose colorful fruits such as berries, cherries, and citrus fruits, which are high in vitamins, minerals, and phytochemicals with strong antioxidant capabilities. These fruits can be eaten fresh as a snack, mixed into salads, or baked into desserts for a naturally sweet and nutritious treat.

Include a variety of vegetables, such as spinach, kale, tomatoes, and sweet potatoes, which include antioxidants including vitamin beta-carotene, and lycopene. These vegetables can be eaten raw in salads, roasted as side dishes, or mixed into soups and sauces for added flavor and nutrients.

Consume nuts and seeds such as almonds, walnuts, chia seeds, and flaxseeds, which are high in omega-3 fatty acids and other antioxidants that promote heart and pancreas health. Sprinkle them on salads, yogurt, or porridge, or mix them into baked goods and granola for extra crunch and nutrition.

Experiment with antioxidant-rich herbs and spices like turmeric, ginger, cinnamon, and oregano, which add flavor and aroma to recipes while also providing anti-inflammatory and immune-boosting properties. Use them liberally in marinades, sauces, and seasoning blends to improve both the taste and nutritional value of meals.

By including a range of antioxidant-rich items in your diet, you can enjoy delectable meals while also improving your overall health and well-being, especially if you have chronic pancreatitis.

Anti-inflammatory Spices & Herbs

Individuals with chronic pancreatitis can benefit from introducing anti-inflammatory spices and herbs into their diet to help alleviate symptoms, reduce inflammation, and promote overall pancreatic health. These savory additions not only improve the taste of foods but also provide a number of health benefits.

Turmeric's main ingredient, curcumin, is known for its significant anti-inflammatory qualities. Incorporate turmeric into curries, soups, and stir-fries to add flavor and health benefits.

Ginger is another potent anti-inflammatory spice that helps relieve digestive discomfort and improve gastrointestinal health. Grated ginger can be used in smoothies, teas, and marinades, as well as sauces and dressings, providing a spicy flavor.

Cinnamon not only provides warmth and sweetness to foods, but it also helps to control blood sugar and prevent inflammation. Sprinkle cinnamon on muesli, yogurt, or baked goods for a tasty and nutritious boost.

Garlic and onions contain sulfur compounds, which have anti-inflammatory and immune-boosting qualities. Add minced garlic and chopped onions to sauces, soups, and stir-fries to enhance flavor and aid digestive health.

Herbs like rosemary, thyme, and oregano include antioxidants and anti-inflammatory substances that can benefit pancreatic function. Season roasted vegetables, grilled meats, and marinades with these aromatic herbs to boost flavor and nutrition.

By introducing anti-inflammatory spices and herbs into your cooking, you can enjoy delectable meals while also improving digestive comfort and general pancreatic health, especially if you have chronic pancreatitis.

CHAPTER SIX
Cooking Techniques that Preserve Nutrients

When treating chronic pancreatitis, it is critical to prioritize cooking methods that preserve nutritional value while also improving flavor and digestibility. You can keep critical vitamins, minerals, and antioxidants in your meals by using moderate cooking techniques and avoiding high temperatures and additional fats.

Steaming is a gentle cooking method that helps vegetables maintain their inherent flavors, colors, and nutrients without adding additional fats or oils. Simply set the vegetables in a steamer basket over simmering water and cook until tender-crisp for a nutritious and tasty side.

Poaching is another low-heat cooking method for retaining the moisture and tenderness of proteins such as chicken, fish, and eggs. By boiling meals in tasty broths or stocks, you may add rich flavor while keeping them moist and simple to digest.

Roasting vegetables and proteins at moderate temperatures allows them to caramelize and create rich flavors while avoiding excessive browning or charring. To improve the flavor of ingredients while retaining their nutritious value, apply a little coating of olive oil and seasonings.

Grilling is a popular cooking method that adds a smoky flavor and char marks to foods without the need for additional fats or oils. Choose lean cuts of meat, poultry, or fish then marinade them in fragrant herbs, spices, and citrus juices to enhance flavor and softness.

Stir-frying is the fast cooking of small pieces of ingredients in a hot skillet with little oil, keeping their texture and nutritional value.

To produce vibrant and healthy stir-fry dishes, use high-quality oils such as olive or avocado oil and a variety of colorful veggies.

By using cooking methods that maintain the natural goodness of products, you can enjoy delectable and nutritious meals while improving your overall health and well-being, especially if you have chronic pancreatitis.

Tips for Meal Planning and Leftovers.

Effective meal planning is critical for those with chronic pancreatitis because it ensures a balanced diet that promotes pancreatic health while reducing symptoms and discomfort. By following these meal-planning techniques and making good use of leftovers, you can expedite your cooking process and enjoy tasty and nutritious meals all week.

Begin by planning a weekly meal plan that includes a range of nutrient-dense foods such as lean proteins, whole grains, fruits, veggies, and healthy fats. Take into account your dietary preferences, any food sensitivities or allergies, and any specific advice from your doctor.

Preparing items ahead of time will save you time and energy during the week. Wash, chop, and portion fruits and vegetables, prepare grains and legumes, and marinate proteins ahead of time to simplify meal preparation and cooking.

Make use of leftovers by reusing them in new dishes or including them in future dinners. For example, roast additional veggies to serve with salads, soups, or grain bowls, or use leftover cooked chicken or fish to make sandwiches, wraps, or stir-fries.

Purchase high-quality storage containers to properly store leftovers and meal preparation components in the refrigerator or freezer.

Label containers with the date and contents to keep track of what has to be used and reduce food waste.

Experiment with batch cooking and freezer-friendly dishes that can be prepared in big quantities and portioned for later meals. Soups, stews, casseroles, and grain-based salads are all wonderful batch-cooking alternatives that can be readily reheated to provide quick and filling dinners.

By adding these strategies to your meal planning routine, you may simplify the cooking process, reduce food waste, and ensure that delicious and nutritious meals are always available, especially if you have chronic pancreatitis.

Healthy Sides and Snacks: Fuel Your Day Right

When dealing with chronic pancreatitis, it's critical to nourish your body with nutritious foods that provide prolonged energy and promote overall health. Including nutritious sides and snacks in your daily meals will help you maintain stable blood sugar levels, manage your weight, and reduce inflammation.

Healthy Side Dishes to Complement Any Meal

Side dishes are essential for balancing a meal's nutritional balance. For people with chronic pancreatitis, choosing nutrient-dense sides is very crucial. Consider adding colorful vegetables like leafy greens, broccoli, carrots, and bell peppers, which are high in vitamins, minerals, and antioxidants. Roasting or boiling vegetables with a splash of olive oil and a sprinkling of herbs can improve their flavor without adding excess fats or sugars. Whole grains, such as quinoa, brown rice, and whole wheat couscous, can also deliver fiber and important nutrients, thereby improving digestive health and satiety.

Snack Options for On-the-Go Nutrition:

People suffering from chronic pancreatitis must keep their blood sugar levels steady throughout the day. On-the-go snacks should be convenient, portable, and healthful. Consider fresh fruit, unsalted nuts, and seeds, Greek yogurt, or whole-grain crackers with hummus. These snacks contain carbohydrates, protein, and healthy fats, providing sustained energy and satisfaction between meals. Preparing snack packs or carrying healthy snacks in your luggage will help you fight the temptation to eat less nutritious foods when you're away from home.

Low-Carb Alternatives for Guilt-Free Eating:

Managing carbohydrate intake may help some people with chronic pancreatitis control their blood sugar levels and symptoms. Low-carb snacks can satisfy appetites while preventing blood glucose increases. Consider serving sliced cucumber or bell pepper with hummus, hard-boiled eggs, or turkey lettuce wraps. These snacks are low in carbohydrates but high in protein, fiber, and important nutrients, making them ideal for guilt-free snacking.

Snacks Packed with Antioxidants for Long-Lasting Energy

Antioxidants help to reduce inflammation and protect cells from free radical damage. Incorporating antioxidant-rich snacks into your diet can improve your overall health and wellness. Mixed berries, dark chocolate bars, or a handmade trail mix with nuts, seeds, and dried fruit are all great options. These snacks include a high concentration of antioxidants, vitamins, and minerals, enabling sustained energy and vigor throughout the day.

While snacking can be beneficial in controlling chronic pancreatitis, portion control is necessary to avoid overeating and maintain a healthy weight. Choose single-serving portions or pre-portioned foods to avoid mindless snacking. Pay attention to hunger signs and try to satisfy your cravings without becoming overly full. Incorporating protein and fiber-rich foods into snacks can also increase feelings of fullness and help to reduce overeating between meals. Remember to stay hydrated by drinking water throughout the day, as thirst is sometimes confused with hunger.

Individuals who incorporate these concepts into a Chronic Pancreatitis Management Diet

Cookbook will have access to a choice of excellent and healthy side meals and snacks that will meet their dietary demands and overall health goals. These recipes and recommendations, which range from nutrient-dense sides to easy on-the-go snacks, can help people with chronic pancreatitis maintain a healthy diet while efficiently managing their disease.

Sweet Treats: Indulge Without Guilt

Sweet sweets can bring comfort and joy, especially for people who have chronic pancreatitis. However, the concern of exacerbating symptoms often causes individuals to feel guilty about eating desserts. This portion of the Chronic Pancreatitis Management Diet Cookbook seeks to help readers fulfill their sweet tooth without sacrificing their health.

Dessert Recipes that will not aggravate symptoms

Creating dessert recipes for those with chronic pancreatitis necessitates a careful selection of components that are mild on the pancreas. These recipes focus on foods that are low in fat, sugar, and other irritants while yet providing delicious flavors and sensations. From fruity pleasures to creamy classics, every dish is designed to satisfy without exacerbating symptoms.

Low-Carb Options to Satisfy Your Sweet Tooth

Individuals with chronic pancreatitis must manage their carbohydrate intake since high-carb foods strain the pancreas and cause discomfort. This section includes low-carb desserts that are both delicious and gratifying. These recipes provide guilt-free enjoyment while keeping blood sugar levels under control by using alternative sweeteners and fiber-rich foods.

Antioxidant-Rich Ingredients for Guilt-Free Treats

Antioxidants help to reduce inflammation and protect pancreatic cells from harm. This section emphasizes the necessity of including antioxidant-rich components in dessert dishes to aid healing and overall health. From dark chocolate to berries and almonds, these ingredients not only add flavor but also help to make desserts healthier.

CHAPTER SEVEN
Tips for Mindful Dessert Enjoyment

Mindful eating is vital for those with chronic pancreatitis because it helps them to savor each bite while remaining alert to their body's cues. This section includes practical methods for practicing mindfulness while eating desserts, such as paying attention to portion sizes, chewing gently, and savoring the flavors. Individuals who adopt a mindful approach to dessert consumption can build a healthier relationship with food and better control their symptoms.

Balancing Sweetness and Healthfulness

Finding a balance between sweetness and healthfulness is essential for enjoying sweets while managing chronic pancreatitis. This section delves into ways to lower sugar levels, replace bad fats with nutritional alternatives, and boost flavor profiles with herbs and spices. Individuals can indulge in sweet delights while still meeting their health goals by prioritizing nutrient-dense products and mindful eating techniques.

Ginger Turmeric Smoothie: "Anti-Inflammatory Elixir: Soothing Smoothie with Ginger and Turmeric to Ease Pancreatic Inflammation"

Salmon Avocado Salad: Subtitled "Omega-3 Powerhouse Salad: Fresh Salmon and Creamy Avocado for Pancreatic Health"

Quinoa Vegetable Soup: "Nutrient-Packed Nourishment: Hearty Quinoa Soup with Assorted Vegetables for Pancreatic Support"

Baked Chicken Breast with Steamed Broccoli: Subtitled "Lean Protein Feast: Tender Chicken Breast Paired with Nutrient-Rich Broccoli for Pancreatic Wellness"

Subtitle: "Protein-Packed Perfection: Fluffy Omelette with Spinach and Feta for Pancreatic Health"

Cucumber Avocado Rolls with Tuna: Subtitled "Refreshing Rolls: Cucumber Filled with Creamy Avocado and Tuna for Pancreatic Comfort"

Subtitled "Gentle Pasta Delight: Whole Grain Pasta with Tender Turkey Meatballs for Pancreatic Support"

Banana Oat Pancakes: Subtitled "Morning Comfort Treat: Fluffy Pancakes Made with Oats and Bananas for Pancreatic Ease"

Roasted vegetable medley:

A 30-day meal plan to alleviate symptoms, promote healing, and cultivate optimal pancreatic wellness.

week 1:

Day 1:

Breakfast: Banana oat pancakes.

Snack: Ginger Turmeric Smoothie.

Lunch is Quinoa Vegetable Soup.

Snack: Cucumber Avocado Rolls with Tuna.

Dinner: Baked chicken breast and steamed broccoli.

Continue this pattern for the remainder of the week, integrating various recipes each day while maintaining a balance of nutrients and flavors.

Weeks 2–4:

Alternate recipes to provide variety and choose pancreas-friendly foods.

Prioritise fruits, vegetables, lean proteins, and whole grains over processed foods, saturated fats, and sugary goods.

Stay hydrated with water and herbal tea throughout the day.

Emphasise portion control and listening to the body's instincts to avoid discomfort and improve digestion.

In conclusion, creating a section dedicated to nutritious soups and salads in a chronic pancreatitis treatment diet cookbook necessitates careful product selection, recipe development, and customization possibilities. People can enjoy delicious and gratifying meals while improving their overall health and well-being by focusing on nutrient-dense products, anti-inflammatory components, and gentle cooking methods.

THE END